Simple WAYS TO ENERGIZE

mind, body & soul

Stephanie Tourles

*The mission of Storey Publishing is to serve our customers
by publishing practical information that encourages personal independence
in harmony with the environment.*

Edited by Deborah Balmuth and Karen Levy
Cover design by Wendy Palitz
Cover illustration by Alexandra Eckhardt
Text design and production by Susan Bernier

Printed in the United States by Lake Book

10 9 8 7 6 5 4 3 2 1

ISBN 1-58017-887-1

Introduction

Are you in the throes of a personal energy crisis? If so, you're not alone. Health practitioners report that fatigue, in its many forms, is the most common complaint heard from patients today.

Energy . . . what exactly is it? Most cultures have a name for it — *pneuma* in Greek, *neshamah* in Hebrew, *spiritus* in Latin, *qi* in Chinese, *prana* in Sanskrit, *ki* in Japanese — to refer to mental, physical, and spiritual life energy.

Although you can't physically hold it in your hands, you can see the sun's energy as light, feel it as warmth, and see evidence of it in the life around you. You can hear the invisible energy of thunder during a rainstorm and see purple bolts of lightning through the clouds. The stimulating effects of a nutritious diet can make you more aware of your strength and stamina.

Positive mental energy, too, can be transmitted through a kind word or a thoughtful gesture. Healing energy is conveyed through laying on of hands, Reiki, touch therapy, massage, or simple human contact. Energy can come in the form of inspiration, prayer, meditation, and exercise, as well as from time spent alone, in nature, and with family and friends.

Energy is vital. Energy is power. Along with oxygen and water, we need energy in order to survive and thrive. No matter how much we already have, we can always use more. We need large amounts of energy to get through our hectic schedules and deal with the demands of modern life; sadly, most of us don't have nearly enough of this precious resource. It's an elusive, mysterious force that courses through our being. We know when we have it, and we know when it's flagging.

I hope these energizing tips will help guide you toward recharging your physical body, restoring your spirit, and revitalizing your mental capacities. May you recapture your zest for life, your happiness, your wholeness, and your physical stamina.

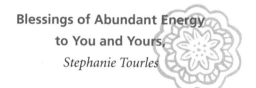

**Blessings of Abundant Energy
to You and Yours,**
Stephanie Tourles

A warm, luxuriant bath is the ultimate way to boost your circulation and balance your energy flow. Pour a tall glass of your favorite beverage, close the door, turn the lights down, put on some background music, light a candle and perhaps some incense, and step in. Feel yourself melt into a pool of pleasure.

Keep a diet diary for a week and write down everything you eat. If your protein intake is less than 20–30 percent of your daily calories, you may feel fatigued. Add a few servings of organic eggs, lean poultry, beef, wild game, fish, whole grains, and beans to your weekly menu.

For a quick energy boost, keep a bottle of peppermint, cypress, eucalyptus, spearmint, or geranium essential oil handy. Place a few drops on a tissue and inhale deeply.

Smooth and Fruity Energy Shake

Start your day with this high-protein, mineral-rich breakfast shake. Makes 2 servings.

- 1 cup calcium-fortified, low-fat plain soy milk
- 1 cup orange juice
- 1 cup raspberries, peaches, strawberries, or pears
- 1 banana
- ½ cup calcium-fortified soft tofu
- 1 scoop soy protein powder
- 1 tablespoon wheat bran or oat bran

Combine all ingredients in a blender and whiz until smooth. Drink immediately.

Your brain's weight is more than 70 percent water. If this proportion drops below a certain point, you'll feel tired and headachy. Drink eight glasses of water daily — more if you're active or if it's hot. Coffee, black tea, and soft drinks don't count. They're diuretics, forcing your kidneys to excrete precious fluid from your body.

Believe in yourself and feel confident that you can achieve anything you set your mind to.

"Live each season as it passes; breathe the air, drink the drink, taste the fruit, and resign yourself to the influences of each."

—Henry David Thoreau

Midafternoon energy slumps are often caused by low blood sugar. Be sure to eat a balanced lunch of lean protein, such as seafood, tofu, tempeh, or chicken, and a complex carbohydrate, such as whole grain bread, tabouli, beans, rice, or potatoes. A pat of butter or olive oil slows digestion, keeping blood sugar stable for several hours.

Follow your heart without asking whether it's okay to do so.

Put an end to a bad relationship.

Did you know that constant sleep deprivation can depress your immune system? We try to pack so much activity into our daily lives that inadequate sleep has hit epidemic levels. Sooner or later you'll pay the price with how you feel, think, and look. Sleep is the best-kept beauty and energy secret around.

"This is the true joy in life, the being used for a purpose recognized by yourself as a mighty one."
— George Bernard Shaw

Green tea — an earthy, natural energizer — is rich in antioxidants and has only one-fifth the caffeine of black tea; it won't make you jittery or stain your teeth.

Avoid eating turkey for lunch. It contains tryptophan, which can cause drowsiness.

Residents in nursing homes love to talk, hold your hand, and relate their life stories. Listening to someone decades older than you can also be a fascinating lesson in history. Take the time to sit and chat for a while and you could make someone very happy.

Mother Nature offers the best medicine for your soul.

Eat a light lunch. Loading up at lunch can leave you feeling tired, especially if you've eaten a carbohydrate-heavy meal of pasta, rice and beans, or bread. Eat a light or moderate lunch and you'll have more energy in the afternoon.

B-vitamin or iron deficiency can lead to an inadequate amount of oxygen in your blood, making you feel lethargic. Even if you think you're eating a healthy diet, you may not be getting enough of these essential nutrients, especially if you're a vegan (strict vegetarian) and/or premenopausal. If a blood test shows a deficiency, follow your doctor's orders by adjusting your diet accordingly. Your energy should soon return.

Negative emotions drain your enthusiasm and zest for life. A positive attitude is refreshing and contagious. Surround yourself with people who are happy and have a strong sense of purpose.

"Spread love everywhere you go: first of all in your own house."

—Mother Teresa

Bright Idea Tea

Spur your creativity and mental awareness with this delicious herbal tea. Makes 4 cups.

1 teaspoon dried ginkgo
1 teaspoon dried hibiscus
1 teaspoon dried lavender
1 teaspoon dried lemon balm
1 teaspoon dried peppermint
1 teaspoon dried spearmint
1 teaspoon dried St.-John's-wort
Pinch stevia to taste

Pour 4 cups of boiling water over the herbs, cover, and steep for 10–20 minutes. Strain and add honey or lemon to taste. Sip throughout the day to keep your mood light and lively. It's particularly good on ice!

Take some bread, crackers, or sunflower seeds to the park to spend some time with your feathered friends. Marvel at the perfection of their feathers and listen to their variety of songs, squawks, and chirps. Notice how light they are on their feet. Then let your energy take flight.

*"**Take a music bath** once or twice a week for a few seasons and you will find that it is to the soul what the water bath is to the body."*

—Oliver Wendell Holmes

Go to bed a little earlier. It's better to get some restful sleep than watch television.

Update your look with a new haircut, makeup colors, or beard or mustache trim.

Even if you're having a bad day, try to find at least one good thing that will bring a smile to your face. It takes more energy to frown, and the act of smiling will boost your energy.

Breathe! Try this simple exercise to help you refocus your energy:

* Stand with your feet shoulder-width apart and place your palms on your lower abdomen.

* Close your eyes and slowly inhale through your nose, gradually expanding your diaphragm. If you're breathing correctly, you will feel your hands move outward.

* Hold for a count of five, then exhale slowly through your mouth.

* Repeat 10 times.

"Those who dare and dare greatly are those who achieve."

—Anonymous

Studies reveal that the more social connections you have, the better your overall health.

Balance your energy fields. Polarity therapy is a holistic approach to healing that aims to balance the body's energy systems. Negative thoughts, pain, tension, stress, and environmental factors contribute to restricted energy flow. Polarity therapy gently manipulates your muscles to unblock energy flow and rebalance your body.

Reiki, which means "universal life energy," is a Japanese healing therapy. The vital energy of the universe is channeled through the practitioner to remove energy blockages and revitalize your body on subtle levels that promote wholeness, harmony, and balance.

Based on the theory of acupuncture, acupressure stimulates special points on the body to help relieve pain and boost energy without needles.

Wake up! Need a bit of afternoon stimulation? Falling asleep after lunch? A shot of oxygen is what you need. Perform this exercise to pump more of this life-sustaining element through your body:

* Stand with your feet shoulder-width apart and place your arms straight out in front of you.
* Slowly do a deep knee bend.
* Squeeze your buttocks on the way back up.
* Repeat 10 times.

Did you know that something as simple as boredom can bring on chronic fatigue?

Shrimp, scallops, clams, crab, abalone, lobster, snails, crayfish, oysters, conch, and prawns increase energy, ease tension, and stabilize moods. Eat two servings per week.

Stimulating Herbal Bath

This herbal bath will invigorate your skin as it rejuvenates your senses.

1 cup fresh or ½ cup dried rosemary, lemon verbena, or sage

1 cup Epsom salts
2 teaspoons olive or sweet almond oil

1. Pour 1 quart of boiling water over the herbs, cover, and steep for 30 minutes. Strain and pour into the bathwater.
2. Add the Epsom salts and oil. Blend well.

The more challenging the situation, the more intrigued you become. Find something challenging to do today!

If you wake up feeling groggy and sluggish, begin your day with some gentle stretching exercises to get your blood and oxygen flowing.

Treat your feet. Wooden footsie rollers come in all shapes and sizes. The kind with raised ridges are both stimulating and relaxing. If you don't have a footsie roller, a wooden rolling pin can be used in a pinch. Simply place the footsie roller or rolling pin on the floor, bear down comfortably, and roll your entire foot back and forth. Repeat, concentrating on your arches, for 5 to 10 minutes per foot.

Peppermint Pizzazz Tea

Intensify the potency of your peppermint tea with this energizing zing.

2 tbsp. fresh or 1 tbsp. dried peppermint
1–2 drops peppermint essential oil

1. Pour 1 cup of boiling water over the herbs. Cover and steep for 10 minutes. Strain.
2. Add the peppermint essential oil. Sip the tea slowly as you inhale the invigorating steam.

Try to exercise outside to help oxygenate your cells with fresh air and facilitate the removal of waste products through your skin. Exercise improves cardiovascular fitness, endurance, and energy. If you live in a city, try to find a park in which to exercise. If city streets, with their attendant pollution, are your only outdoor option, exercising in a gym may be a better alternative.

Point and flex. This is a great exercise to rev up the circulation in your legs and put the spring back in your step.
* Take your shoes off; sit on the floor with your legs stretched out in front of you and your palms facing down at your sides.
* Point your toes as hard as you can and hold for 5 seconds, then flex your feet as hard as you can and hold for 5 seconds.
* Repeat 10 times.

"The people who live long are those who long to live."

—Anonymous

Try this simple massage technique when you're feeling frazzled. Hold your foot in one hand and grasp your big toe with the thumb and index finger of your other hand. Slowly and firmly pull on your toe, starting at the base and sliding your fingers to the top. Gently squeeze and roll the toe between your thumb and index finger. Repeat on the remaining toes, then switch feet.

Nourish your creative spirit.

Ten to 15 minutes of unprotected exposure to sunlight several times a week is essential for healthy skin and bones. Sun exposure also energizes your body.

Find creative ways to integrate family time with exercise. If you have children, don't just be a bystander at the playground — climb the jungle gym or play softball. Push a jogging stroller. Get a baby seat for your bicycle or sign up for swimming lessons together at the YMCA.

Lemon Lover's Lift

This herbal tea blend will help recharge your mental powers. Makes 2 cups.

  2 teaspoons dried lemon balm leaves
  2 teaspoons dried lemon verbena leaves
  2 teaspoons dried lemongrass

1. Pour 2 cups of boiling water over the herbs, cover, and steep for 5 to 10 minutes. Strain.
2. Add a squirt of fresh lemon juice, orange juice, honey, or maple syrup to taste.

A good heart-to-heart conversation can lighten your mood, ease your worries, and restore your connection to others.

There's no better way to energize your body, mind, and spirit than by taking care of yourself.

"Never esteem anything of advantage to you that will make you break your word or lose your self-respect."
—Marcus Aurelius Antoninus

For a cool, nutritious, energizing snack, try frozen seedless grapes. To prepare, pluck the grapes off the stems, place them on a cookie sheet with raised edges, and put them in the freezer for an hour. Eat immediately or store in a freezer bag for later.

Get a pet. Studies show that pet owners live healthier, happier, less stressful lives. Dogs will help you get more exercise. Pets make great companions and live-in psychotherapists, too.

"Health is something we do for ourselves, *not something that is done to us; a journey rather than a destination; a dynamic, holistic, and purposeful way of living."*

—Dr. Elliott Dacher

To boost your brain power, eat high-protein snacks, such as peanut butter, sesame butter, or cottage cheese.

Maintain a positive attitude. Negativity affects your mood, job performance, physical appearance, and health. Your mood is contagious to those around you, too.

Energizing Bath Oil

This massage oil can be used when you need physical and mental stimulation.

- 1 tablespoon grape-seed, hazelnut, jojoba, or sweet almond oil
- 2 drops each of eucalyptus, peppermint, and rosemary essential oils

Blend the ingredients. Add the oil to your bath while the tap is running or use as a massage oil after a bath or shower.

Nothing is more cheerful than colorful flowering plants. Select a few long-lasting and plentiful bloomers and put them in the places where you spend the most time.

Stimulate your brain. Don't allow yourself to become bored with life.

The next time you go on vacation, collect colorful seashells, stones, or other mementos. Fill an inexpensive, clear glass lamp base with your prize collection. You'll be reminded of your trip every time you turn on the lamp.

Buy flowering bulbs for the dead of winter. Hyacinth, paper-white, daffodil, and tulip bulbs are perfect for "forcing." Insert the bulbs root-side down into an inch of white gravel, shells, or marbles in a shallow dish; add extra gravel to mid-bulb height. Set the pot in a bright, sunny window. Water with liquid flowering-plant fertilizer and keep moist until flowering is complete.

If your get-up-and-do-it got up and took a hike a long time ago, try listening to inspirational or motivational tapes while you drive.

Eat fresh, whole, unprocessed foods. Avoid empty-calorie, chemical-laden junk foods. They do nothing but satisfy a temporary craving. Real food satisfies your soul and truly nourishes your body.

To increase your energy, shower in water that's approximately body temperature for 2 to 3 minutes, then lower the temperature to very cool for 15 to 30 seconds. Repeat twice.

"I was always looking outside myself for strength and confidence but it comes from within. It is there all the time."
—Anna Freud

Rediscover the joys of an imaginative journey through reading. Keep a selection of soul-nourishing books at your bedside.

Whatever your passion in life, do it with gusto!

Learn to cross-country ski. If you feel cooped up and lethargic in the winter, cross-country skiing is the perfect antidote. It's one of the best exercises for overall body toning, and your lungs get a workout in the invigorating, chilly air.

For a rejuvenating foot treatment, blend 6 drops of peppermint essential oil with 1 tablespoon of sweet almond oil. Massage your clean feet with the mixture for 15 minutes. Then put on socks to absorb the excess oil and condition your feet all day.

Kick off your shoes and walk barefoot in the grass. Let the warm, soft earth caress your feet.

Many people think that yoga is for people who can't do strenuous exercise. That assumption couldn't be further from the truth. Yoga strengthens and tones your muscles and joints by using your own body weight for resistance. It also builds balance, coordination, and stamina.

Cook a spicy meal for breakfast. Add hot salsa to your scrambled eggs, jalapeño jelly to your toast, or a little cayenne, cinnamon, and nutmeg to your oatmeal. Spicy foods stimulate your metabolism and awaken your senses for the day ahead.

Enhance the romance. Place several scented candles of varying heights in front of a mirror. Light them for a romantic effect. They will scent the air, and you can watch the flames flicker and dance.

Meal in a Cup

Fortify your mind and body with this nutritious blend of vitamins, minerals, carbohydrates, protein, and fiber. Makes 1 serving.

1 cup plain, low-fat yogurt or fortified soy yogurt

¼ cup almonds, raisins, or granola

½ cup ripe fruit

1 teaspoon honey or maple syrup (optional)

Combine all ingredients and blend well. Eat immediately.

Enhance your energy level and ability to concentrate by practicing deep breathing.

* Close your eyes.
* Breathe in deeply through your nose and hold for a count of eight.
* Exhale completely through your mouth.
* Repeat ten times.

Give your body the brush off. For an invigorating morning ritual, try dry brushing to stimulate your circulation and shed your snake skin. Dry brushing is performed on dry skin — not oiled, not damp — but dry, before-you-shower skin. Use a natural-fiber brush to gently massage your body, except your face and breasts, for 5 to 10 minutes. Never scrub until you're red.

Communicate with nature. Explore the nearby woods, enjoy a garden, or just sit outside on the grass and appreciate the sights, sounds, and smells.

Clear your head. Take a day off and spend it antiquing, visiting a museum exhibit you've been longing to see, going to flea markets, or picnicking in a public garden. A change of scenery will do you good.

The lovely, floral fragrance of lavender essential oil can soothe your soul without sapping your energy. To enhance concentration and promote mental clarity, place a drop on your wrist, the palms of your hands, or the nape of your neck and breathe deeply.

"Let no one ever come to you without leaving better and happier."

—Mother Teresa

Reconnect with loved ones. Write a letter to a long-lost friend or relative.

Do something that will make you feel good about yourself; buy yourself a special treat or take a day off from work and do exactly what you want.

Add Life to Your Tresses

Stimulate your scalp as you add shine and moisture to your hair. Makes 20 treatments.

- 4 tablespoons jojoba oil
- 1 tablespoon 80-proof vodka
- 2 teaspoons lavender essential oil
- 1 teaspoon basil essential oil
- 1 teaspoon geranium essential oil
- 1 teaspoon grapefruit essential oil
- 1 teaspoon yarrow essential oil
- 1 teaspoon lemon essential oil

Mix all ingredients together in a dark glass bottle. Shake well before use. Massage 1 teaspoon into your scalp with your fingertips for 3 minutes. Leave on for 1 hour or longer for maximum effect. Wash out with a mild shampoo. Repeat two or three times per week.

Phone a friend. Call someone who needs some cheering up. A bit of laughter and stimulating conversation will do you both good.

Incorporate peanut butter, a high-energy food, into your diet for a perfect on-the-go snack.

Practice self-affirmations every day to keep a positive perspective. Here are some examples:

* I trust myself completely.
* I am a smart and talented go-getter.
* I am calm and relaxed no matter what the circumstances.
* I am at peace.
* I will not worry, no matter what comes my way today.
* I can do anything I set my mind to.

When you're feeling fatigued, try a short nap for about 30 minutes. Don't fall asleep; simply close your eyes and rest. This brief time of stillness rejuvenates your mind and body.

*"**A man becomes** what he thinks about all day long."*

—Ralph Waldo Emerson

Enjoy more soy. Soybeans are touted as today's miracle food — and justifiably so. Abundant in fiber and complex carbohydrates, soybeans have an almost perfect amino acid profile, similar to that of animal protein. They even contain lysine, an amino acid not commonly found in many plant foods. Include tofu, soy protein powder, soy flour, soy nuggets, soybeans, and soy milk in your daily diet.

Sit quietly and listen to your heart; it often gives the best advice.

Surprise your loved one with a special, candlelit dinner and a tempting chocolate dessert.

Eating several small meals throughout the day rather than two or three large ones keeps your sugar level stable and prevents mood swings and headaches. It also regulates your appetite and ensures a steady stream of nutrients throughout the day. Digesting small meals requires less energy than digesting large ones. Thanksgiving dinner makes you sleepy — remember?

"The strongest principle of growth lies in human choice."

—George Eliot

There is a useful old adage that says "one must say goodbye before one says hello." Letting go is an act of strength and courage. It helps healing begin, frees you of the weight of the past, lightens the present, and opens doors to a new future.

Eat five to ten servings per day of the following fruits and vegetables. They're low in calories and high in energizing nutrients.

* Berries: Grapes, blackberries, blueberries, cranberries, strawberries, and boysenberries
* Fruits: Apples, apricots, peaches, bananas, pears, kiwis, grapefruits, lemons, oranges, and plums
* Vegetables: Loose-leaf and romaine lettuce, spinach, broccoli, Brussels sprouts, kale, carrots, tomatoes, red peppers, string beans, cabbage, onions, potatoes, and celery
* Melons: Cantaloupe, watermelon, honeydew, and Crenshaw

Be the kind of friend who lends a helping hand.

Strengthen the bond with your loved one by creating more intimacy together.

"Let's be grateful *for those who give us happiness; they are the charming gardeners who make our soul bloom."*

—Marcel Proust

Upbeat, optimistic people are more likely to be healthy, energetic, and successful. A Swedish study of senior citizens found that mental health was an even stronger predictor of longevity than physical health was.

Wear red, orange, or yellow to brighten your mood.

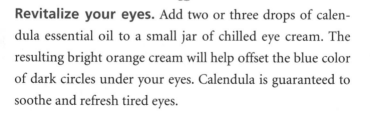

Revitalize your eyes. Add two or three drops of calendula essential oil to a small jar of chilled eye cream. The resulting bright orange cream will help offset the blue color of dark circles under your eyes. Calendula is guaranteed to soothe and refresh tired eyes.

Power-Packed Vegetarian Soup

This delicious soup is rich in antioxidants, minerals, and fiber and packs a nutritional wallop. Makes 6 quarts.

1½ quarts low-sodium vegetable juice
5 cups water or vegetable stock
3½ cups crushed tomatoes
1 package dried onion soup mix
12 cloves garlic, peeled
8 stalks celery, chopped into 2-inch pieces
4 medium white onions, peeled and quartered
1 medium green cabbage, chopped into 2-inch chunks
1 large green pepper, chopped into 2-inch chunks
1 habanero pepper, stem and seeds removed
1 large red pepper, chopped into 2-inch chunks

1. In a 6-quart stockpot, heat the vegetable juice, water or vegetable stock, crushed tomatoes, and onion soup mix.

2. Grind the garlic, celery, onion, cabbage, and peppers in batches in a food processor until almost minced. Add to soup stock. Mix well.

3. Cover, reduce the heat to a simmer, and cook for 2 hours, stirring occasionally.

Touch therapy: the benefits go both ways. Touching another person sets up an exchange of healing energy, which results in a greater sense of well-being for both of the people involved. Research shows that hospital and nursing home patients experience quicker recovery when receiving touch therapy.

Shovel some snow. If you're a northerner, throw away your snow blower and pick up a shovel. The lunging, lifting, and heaving deliver an intense workout, and shoveling gets you outdoors, too. You may even develop an appreciation for the beauty of snow.

Get in shape and save money by mowing your lawn yourself. Using a push mower rather than a power mower provides all-over body conditioning.

Reduce or eliminate high-fat dairy products, red meat, refined flour, and sugary foods from your diet. They sap your energy and increase your risk of developing cancer, arthritis, osteoporosis, heart disease, bowel problems, high blood pressure, and diabetes. Eat a wide variety of whole foods as close to their natural state as possible. Unprocessed foods generally contain more nutrients, are void of questionable additives, and cost less than their processed peers.

Make lunchtime work for you. Use your lunchtime to go outside, breathe deeply, and move your body. It's a terrific way to recharge yourself so you'll be at your peak productivity level in the afternoon.

Buy a book of affirmations and carry it with you. Read it throughout the day to lift your spirits and instill confidence.

For a healthful, nutrient-dense snack, grab a handful of raw walnuts or Brazil nuts, or chop them and add them to your salads in lieu of croutons.

You are what you drink. Try to avoid coffee, black tea, soda, alcohol, and refined juices. Coffee and black tea are addictive stimulants. They stain your teeth and leave you dehydrated. Soda is loaded with chemicals and phosphoric acid, which decays tooth enamel and leaches calcium from your bones. Alcohol damages your liver and kidneys and acts as a powerful diuretic. The excessive processing of refined juices removes their life force.

Look forward to something. Plan a vacation, getaway weekend, or fun day trip. When stress strikes, recall the event you've planned for the near future.

Life's best lessons are learned from life's problems — these are your teachers.

"The best way to predict your future is to create it."
—Peter Drucker

We are a society of shallow, tidal breathers. Constantly rushing around in a frenzy, we rarely utilize our full lung capacity, resulting in a constant state of fatigue. Most of us breathe from the upper portion of our lungs without expanding our diaphragm and taking a really deep, energizing and oxygenating breath. Be aware of your breathing habits and try to focus on breathing properly, which will energize your body and mind.

Learn to listen to the messages your body gives you.

Eucalyptus Inhalation

Eucalyptus essential oil has a camphorlike aroma that stimulates mental function.

    4 cups water
    6 drops eucalyptus oil

1. Boil the water, remove it from the heat, and add the oil.
2. Drape a towel over your head and the pot and inhale the vapors for 10 minutes. Be sure to keep your eyes closed.

*"**Without this playing with fantasy** no creative work has ever yet come to birth."*

—Carl Gustav Jung

Visualization: create scenes in your mind of happiness, health, and success. Fill in the details with sounds, colors, and scents. Pull up these images whenever you need a boost.

Flaxseed oil is high in omega-3 fatty acids, which help fight fatigue, dry skin, itchy scalp, dandruff, arthritis pain, allergies, immune deficiencies, and constipation while improving eyesight and color perception. Consume 2 tablespoons daily. Ground flaxseeds are good sprinkled over salads, too.

Leave your car in the garage and dust off that old bike. Use it for all your short errands.

Kick up your legs. You don't have to be a Las Vegas showgirl to have long, lean legs and tight buttocks. Place one hand on a sturdy chair, stand straight and tall, and kick your right leg as high as you possibly can without slouching or bending at the waist. Do 10 kicks, then change legs. Work up to 100 kicks per leg daily. This is a great cardiovascular exercise that jump-starts your energy, as well.

Blue-green algae is rich in omega-6 fatty acids, beta-carotene, and trace minerals. It combats fatigue, arthritis, psoriasis, acne, and eczema. Take 2 teaspoons daily.

Rev up your posterior circulation. Does your job require that you sit down all day? Feel like your fanny is spreading? Then learn to do isometric squeezes to stimulate circulation in your lower half. These can be performed anywhere, and no one else will know you're doing them. Squeeze your buttocks as hard as you can, hold for 5 seconds, and release. Repeat as many times as you can as often as possible.

Train for a local 5k or 10k fun run or benefit walk in your community. You may not break any speed records, but it will feel great to accomplish a goal and to be among others who have done the same.

Carbohydrates, organic compounds that furnish a large percentage of energy, are needed in a healthy diet. Foods high in carbohydrates include beans, fruits, rice, whole grain cereals, pasta, corn, potatoes, and bread. During digestion, carbohydrates are broken down into energy-producing compounds.

"Life is a daring adventure or nothing."

—Helen Keller

Stimulating Ginger Tea

Ginger tea is recommended for flagging energy, colds, flu, motion sickness, and gas pain.

1. Pour 1 cup of boiling water over ½ ounce of grated, fresh gingerroot.
2. Cover and steep for 15 minutes.
3. Strain and add honey and lemon juice for a unique, natural "ginger ale" taste.

Be the kind of friend who laughs at all jokes, even if they're not that funny.

Here are two yoga postures that are perfect for easing into your day.

* Start on all fours in the "table" position.
* Inhale slowly, raise your head, and gently arch your back as you push your tailbone up until you are in the "cat" position.
* Exhale slowly, round your spine, push your hands into the floor, roll your tailbone down, and pull in your belly.
* Repeat several times.

"You ask me what I came into the world to do. I came to live out loud."

—Emile Zola

Splash cold water on your face and run your hands and wrists under the cold water tap.

For a quick shot of energy, stand up and do this exercise: Bend over at the waist and hang your head down so that your hands are touching your toes (if possible) and you're looking at your knees. Relax your upper body. Hold this position for several seconds, then slowly rise.

Get rid of clutter. Lighten your load. Unclutter your closet, purse, office, bureau, garage, attic, and basement. Hold a tag sale or take everything to a local charity.

"You just can't beat the person who never gives up."
—George "Babe" Ruth

Know your limits. Learn to say "no" more often to demanding friends, family, and co-workers who seem to sap every ounce of energy you have to spare.

Clean up your emotional life by forgiving someone who has done you wrong.

Enjoy the little pleasures. Are you so busy that you overlook life's little pleasures? Living at breakneck speed puts you on a wild roller coaster ride and makes you feel physically exhausted and spiritually frazzled. Set aside time for yourself, on a regular basis, to revel in the small, daily pleasures.

Call a good massage therapist and book a full-body massage. Your mind, body, and spirit will be revitalized.

Brewer's Yeast Mask

This mask is recommended for those with normal to oily skin. It helps chase away a pasty winter complexion and removes dull, dry skin buildup. Makes 1 treatment.

1 tablespoon brewer's yeast
1 tablespoon milk or water

1. Combine the ingredients to form a smooth paste. You may need more or less liquid, depending on the brand of yeast you use.
2. Spread the paste onto your clean face in a thin layer.
3. Let the paste dry, then rinse with cool water.

This mask may tingle as it dries. This is normal. If it starts to sting, rinse it off immediately and apply a good moisturizer.

Green leafy vegetables, such as collard greens and spinach, are packed with folate, vitamins A and C, magnesium, potassium, and calcium. Eat a cup or more per week.

Poor posture is hard on your spine. It compresses your lungs, depriving your body of oxygen, and accelerates gravity's effects on your facial contours. To improve your posture, walk around with a book balanced on your head. Learn to adopt this posture routinely.

" . . . If one advances confidently in the direction of his dreams, and endeavors to live the life which he has imagined, he will meet with a success unexpected in common hours."

—Henry David Thoreau

Raise your metabolic rate — the rate at which you burn calories. Spices such as cardamom, ginger, cinnamon, onions, chili pepper, black pepper, garlic, and hot mustard help your body burn calories faster by producing internal heat. As a bonus, spicy foods stimulate circulation.

Indulge your chocolate craving. Chocolate increases the levels of the mood-boosting hormones dopamine and serotonin in your brain and is a source of phenylethylamine, an antidepressant. Chocolate tastes great, too, so eating it stimulates the pleasure centers in your brain.

Get rid of so-called "friends" who are negative or who bring you down.

"Every day is a birthday; every moment of it is new to us; we are born again, renewed for fresh work and endeavor."
—Issac Watts

Sing out! Singing draws more oxygen into your body, enhances mental clarity, and banishes fatigue.

Your feet are more sensitive and receptive to touch than your hands, because they contain a wealth of nerve endings. Sit on the edge of the bathtub and alternately blast your feet with cold and hot water at 10-second intervals.

Refresh your senses. Scented geraniums come in many fragrant varieties, such as rose, mint, spicy ginger, cinnamon, lemon, orange, peach, and strawberry. Put one on your desk or bedside table near a sunny window and gently rub the leaves between your fingers when you need a lift.

Store your astringent or toner in the refrigerator. After cleansing your face, enjoy an invigorating rinse by splashing cool toner over your face and chest. Your pores will look temporarily smaller and your complexion more refined.

Ginkgo biloba — a popular supplement — boosts circulation to the brain, enhancing memory and alertness.

Rosemary for remembrance. This pungently fragrant culinary and medicinal herb is a universal favorite for boosting memory and mental performance. Rosemary is available in the forms of essential oil, capsules, tincture, or loose-leaf tea and may also be used fresh or dried in your favorite dishes.

Value yourself as much as you expect others to value you.

Keep a journal . . . or a memory book. It's a great way to download the day's activities, reflect on the decisions you've made, and ponder the future. It's a soul-enriching experience to go back and relive your life's journey.

Laughter makes you feel good, makes your skin glow, and stimulates circulation of blood and oxygen throughout your entire body. It also "massages" your internal organs. Go see a funny movie or play, read an amusing book, watch a comedy on televesion, tickle your children, tell some jokes, or play with your pet.

Try this yogic breathing technique when you need a quick energy boost.

* Sit down and close your eyes.
* Press your finger over your right nostril and inhale deeply and slowly through your left nostril. Exhale through your mouth.
* Press your finger over your left nostril and inhale deeply and slowly through your right nostril. Exhale through your mouth.
* Alternate breathing through each nostril five times.

Take a hike . . . or a walk. March in place. Climb some stairs. Jump rope. Do a few squats or high kicks. Aerobic exercise, even for just 5 minutes, increases your energy level.

"Cheerfulness and content are great beautifiers and are famous preservers of youthful looks."
—Charles Dickens

Research has shown that people who eat breakfast have higher metabolic rates than people who skip this vitally important meal.

If you're desk bound all day, try to get up and walk around for a few minutes every hour. Take the stairs at the other end of the building, use the copy machine in another office, or use the restroom on another floor.

Go for a swim at the local YMCA, backyard pool, lake, or ocean. You'll feel powerful, graceful, and limber from this cooling energizer.

Embrace yourself. Think about what makes you feel attractive, strong, smart, or energetic. Make a list. Recite it to yourself when you need a boost.

Scatter fun minibreaks into your daily routine.

Do you have a particular craft skill that might interest children? If so, volunteer to share your knowledge at a local camp, school, or library. Skills such as basic pottery, sculpting, drawing, painting, jewelry making, weaving, or basket making can be magical for children of all ages.

*"**Develop interest in life** as you see it; in people, things, literature, music — the world is so rich, simply throbbing with rich treasures, beautiful souls and interesting people."*

—Henry Miller

Beans, beans, the magical food . . . the more you eat, the better your mood! It's true: Beans are high in B vitamins, which are mood stabilizers. They're also rich in complex carbohydrates, magnesium, iron, zinc, and fiber. A cup or so a day is recommended.

Your internal clock thrives on consistency, so if you spend your weekends staying up late and sleeping in the next morning, your body perceives this as pseudo jet lag without even setting foot in the airport. Try to establish a regular routine and don't stray from it by more than 30 minutes to an hour.

Pick-Me-Up Tea

Try this tea blend to start your morning on an energetic note or to recharge your stamina during the day. Makes 2 cups.

    2 teaspoons dried ginger mint leaves
    2 teaspoons dried orange mint leaves
    2 teaspoons dried pineapple mint leaves

1. Pour 2 cups of boiling water over the herbs, cover, and steep for 5 to 10 minutes. Strain.
2. Add a squirt of lemon or orange juice and sweetener, if desired.

"Most of us will miss out on life's big prizes: the Pulitzers, the Heismans, the Oscars. But we're all eligible for a pat on the back, a kiss on the cheek, a thumbs-up sign!"
—Barbara Johnson

Cultivate close friendships and renew old ones. They can be a source of strength when times are rough.

Make a list of the past successes in your life. By remembering your accomplishments, you'll have the confidence necessary to achieve even greater ones.

Decide what you want for your future. Stake your claim. Having a goal or vision will give your life direction, purpose, and passion.

"Mindfulness provides a simple but powerful route for getting ourselves unstuck, back in touch with our own wisdom and vitality."

—Jon Kabat-Zinn

"Affirmation of life *is the spiritual act by which man ceases to live unreflectively and begins to devote himself to his life with reverence in order to raise it to its true value."*

—Albert Schweitzer

What we manifest in this life is a reflection of what dwells deep inside us: our values, beliefs, and self-esteem. If we want to renew our lives, we have to change our inner beliefs about our right to happiness and vitality.

Every big change begins with a baby step.

Expand your horizons. Today, do one thing that you've really wanted to do but were afraid to try. Perhaps you've felt too intimidated or too old. Stretch yourself beyond your usual limits.

"One who plants a garden, plants happiness."

—Anonymous

In our modern, hectic society, personal time is frequently shoved aside in an effort to accomplish more at an increasingly frenetic pace. Reclaim your personal time and you'll naturally reclaim your own energy.

Herbal Body Wash

½ cup dried lemon verbena leaves
½ cup uncooked oatmeal
1 small muslin bag

Put the lemon verbena and oatmeal in the muslin bag. Moisten the bag thoroughly with water and rub it over your skin as a moisturizing pick-me-up. These small, fragrant bags also make lovely gifts.

What do you really want? Ask yourself with gentleness and patience, "In my heart of hearts, what do I truly want?" Be still, listen, and honor the answers that come. It may be a while before you hear the truest answer, which often speaks in a very quiet, almost imperceptible voice. This answer may be different from the life you are leading. That's okay. Simply live with this new insight and follow where it beckons.

Cultivate an attitude of gratitude.

Knowledge is power. Empower yourself by reading more books, watching movies, and attending plays. Visit museums, go to seminars, take classes. By expanding your scope of knowledge, you'll enlarge your mental reference library. This knowledge can be drawn on in the future — who knows where it could take you?

Pursue only those things in life that support harmony, balance, inspiration, and spiritual enlightenment.

Drink your greens. Green grasses, such as barley, alfalfa, and wheatgrass, and algae, including spirulina and chlorella, are touted as "superfoods" because they are chock-full of vitamins, minerals, enzymes, and chlorophyll. Available in health food stores in powders, capsules, or tablets that contain either single items or blends of grasses, algae, and herbs, these supplements provide quick energy and the long-lasting benefits of green vegetables.

"Whether you think you can, or think you can't, you're probably right."

—Henry Ford